The Magic of Neem

Margosa to Heal

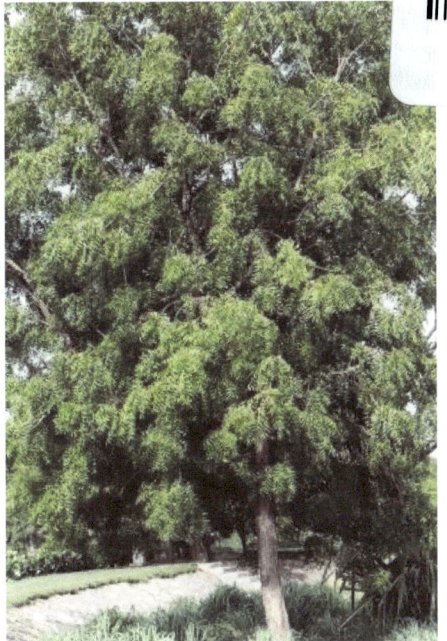

Dueep Jyot Singh

Natural Remedy Series

Mendon Cottage Books

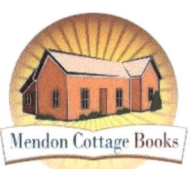

JD-Biz Publishing

Our books are available at

1. Amazon.com
2. Barnes and Noble
3. Itunes
4. Kobo
5. Smashwords
6. Google Play Books

Table of Contents

Introduction

Most of us may have heard the name of an indigenous plant found in the East, – Neem. This is the local name for a plant called Margosa-the Indian Neem. Its scientific name is Azadirachta indica.

This is a long living tree, which has come down in Indian mythology as one of the gifts of the gods, given to the people of *Jambudwipa*- the prehistoric and historic name of the area which consisted of the Indian subcontinent. That is the reason why this plant is worshipped in many ancient traditional rituals of some religious sects in India.

No Indian garden is considered to be complete without a Neem tree growing. The idea is that the grandfather is going to plant the Neem tree, and the future generations up to the seventh generation are going to derive benefit of this plant. That is why the first thing one does when one buys a new house is plant a Neem tree and then plant some other fruit trees like mangoes and lemons.

The Neem tree used to grow wild, but it is now cultivated extensively throughout the land. It is estimated that there are about 138 million Neem trees cultivated by farmers in Neem plantations throughout India. We are not talking about the ones which grow completely wild in the forests and in the woods or in your gardens.

There has been a long mythological history of the Neem, coming down the ages. Let me give you one example. The Neem grown on the outskirts of the village, would be worshipped by ancient villagers, who wanted the friendly spirits living on the Neem to grant them their wishes. That is why, they often fed the Neem with milk or buried copper coins underneath the Neem tree. I do not know who took advantage of the buried coins, but I saw this pattern being followed as an adult, when people got to know about the only Neem tree, in the locality, which happened to have been planted by my grandfather four decades earlier.

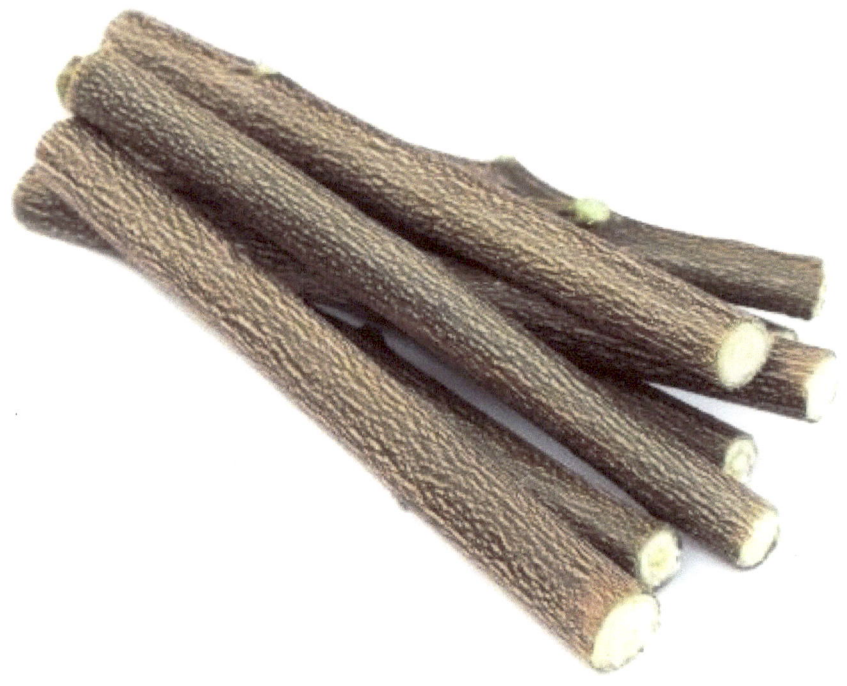

Neem twigs are used as a toothbrush, even today. You break off a twig, chew it to keep your teeth healthy, and then brush your teeth with this chewed portion. It is definitely bitter in taste, but you never will not have to visit a dentist.

A Neem tree needs lots of place to grow, so that is why it is never planted near a wall. That is because within 20 years or so, the roots expand so much that the wall has to be uprooted, thanks to the creeping roots. That is why the Neem tree was always planted in ancient times, outside the village along with the holy "Bel" and other indigenous trees.

Thus, this Neem tree became the focus of everyone's aspirations and they brought their red spangled and embroidered pieces of scarves, to tie on the stem of the Neem tree and some money to bury under it. One fine day, I found a worshiper knocking an iron nail into my poor Neem. That was the outside of enough. Once people began to do that, they would be enough of nails knocked into that poor unprotesting plant for me to hang my whole wardrobe on my Neem tree.

It was time to take care of my Neem, which was my childhood playmate, being the deck of Christopher Columbus's ships or any lonesome eyrie where the intrepid hunter sat while man eating tigers prowled around. Give a child a tree with many branches, and you open up a whole new world of imagination for it! So I needed the help of some friendly ghosts, and spirits which were supposed to live on my dear Neem and grant the wishes of all the superstitious dimwits. What fools these mortals be!

So the very next evening, when I was sitting under the Neem tree, I just looked up and waved, "hi!" Naturally, there was no one around. I continued this activity, for a couple of nights, after looking around very carefully to see that there was no one around. The word went forth. Col. Saheb's granddaughter [*you know, the weird silent one from the jungles of the East where black magic was practiced every hour…*] stood under the Neem and spoke to some things only she could see. She never spoke to them, when there were people around. And she took really good care of the Neem. Could it be that that uncanny female "saw something"? And the Spirits spoke to her?

So within the week, it was official. She did. At night, she sat under the tree, when nobody in his right senses did that at night. She also laughed occasionally to herself. And if one listened very carefully, one heard the jingle of small bells in response. [All right, let me admit it; I had hung up an anklet on one of the branches.]

So one day one of the villagers approached me in fear and trembling. They had heard that I talked to the spirits of the Neem. I gave an insouciant laugh, "You mean my friend Zenaab and her family? They are very happy to live here. Only, they were asking me why you were hurting the poor Neem, by pounding nails into its trunk. " She shivered. I seemed sane. She quavered on," What should we do then? We want something which grants us our wishes."

I said "If you want to tie red scarves, bring long red scarves which can go round the trunk. Do not nail them to the trunk. That is what Zenaab told me to tell you. She also said, that the spirits of the Neem have heard your prayers. Now it is up to you to work towards its fulfillment. Do not just keep expecting the spirits to help you, if you do not do anything towards gaining that goal. "

She went away, deeply impressed. The spirits were good. They were talking sense. This is what comes of being a psychologist and a "showman"!

That Neem tree flourished for another 20 years with plenty of organic manure and plenty of coins buried under its roots. How many of those prayers were fulfilled? Surprisingly enough, a large number of them were fulfilled, because of autosuggestion. The spirits had spoken. They would be obeyed.

So now you know how much this tree is a part of ancient myth and civilization in the East.

But then, there is reason for that happening. Every leaf, branch, seed, and bark of the Neem can be put to use. The seeds are crushed to make Neem oil. They are also used to make natural pesticide, which was the only natural, organic fertilizer and pesticide use in the East, for centuries. So anyone trying to patent this process as something he thought up is going to be laughed out of court.

Neem oil

How do you get Neem oil?

Neem oil is extracted from the seeds. The residual matter left over after the seeds have been crushed and the oil extracted is used as an organic fertilizer.

On the other hand, the leaves of the Neem are used for making herbal teas, and tisanes. The bark is made into a paste with water, to cure skin problems.

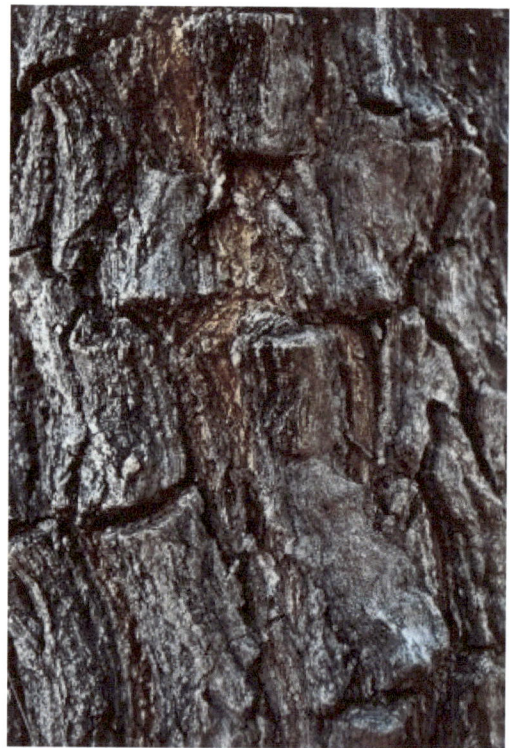

The outer portions of the bark, as well as the inner layer, just under the bark are used in different medical preparations for skin care and other ailments.

Make your Skin Blemish Free

You can also try this beauty treatment to keep your skin blemish free.

Someone suggested whether I would try this remedy – a couple of Neem oil drops to Vaseline, in the winter, if you are using it as a skin moisturizer. To tell you very frankly, Vaseline is petroleum jelly, obtained as the residue when petroleum is refined. It is excellent as a grazing material, but I do not normally use it on my skin. It has gone through some process in which some chemical procedure has occurred.

So instead of petroleum jelly, try, Neem oil mixed with coconut oil, or almond oil, if you want to moisturize your skin. It works wonders!

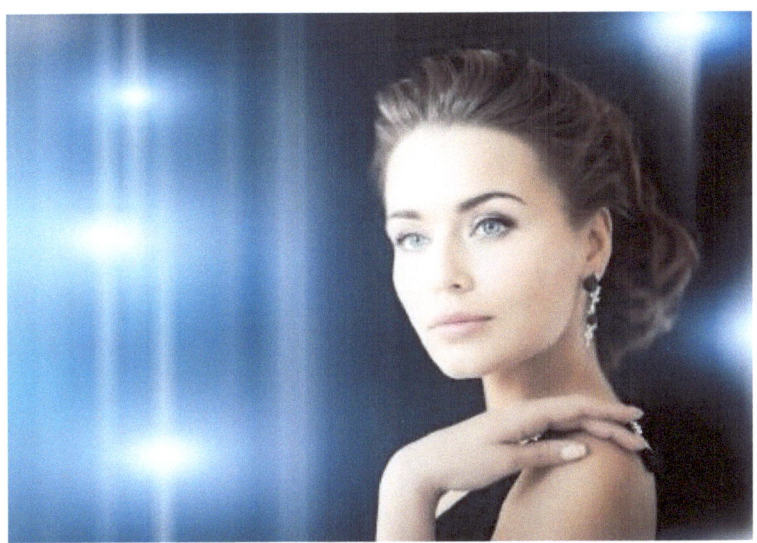

Blemish free and well moisturized skin is a thing of beauty and a joy forever.

How to Grow a Neem

A Neem takes anywhere between 10 to 20 years to grow and flourish. It needs lots of space to grow, so that it can expand in girth. However, it is going to start producing seeds, within 3 to 5 years. The Neem flowers in the summer. The flowers have also been used for centuries for medicinal purposes and in cooking. The seed looks like an unripe green grape. Just like the grape ripening, it is also going to turn yellow when it is totally ripe. These seeds can be collected in bunches.

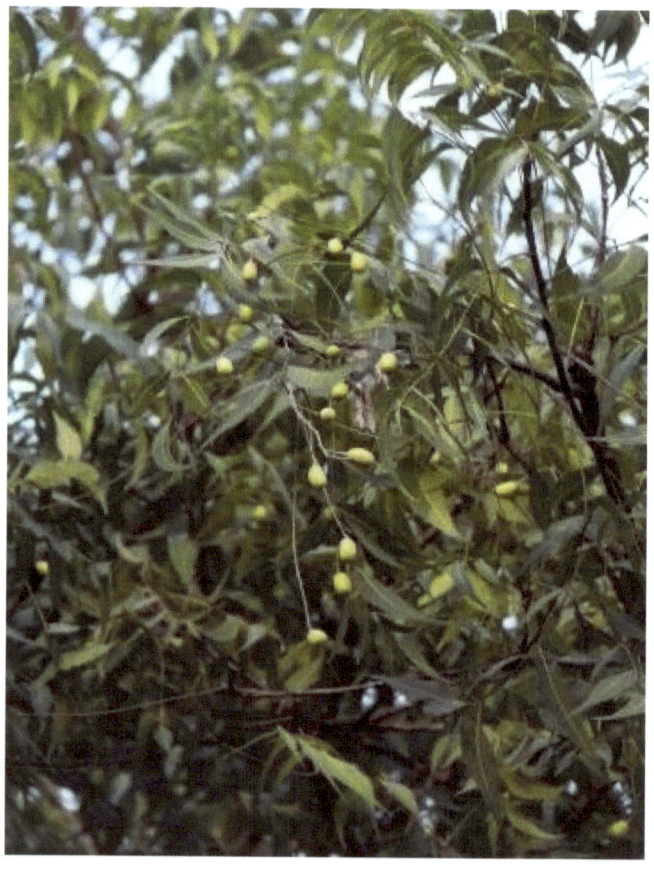

You can grow this plant, from seedlings in your nursery or you can just grow them directly from seeds, planted in the spring. Just pop them in a well-watered and well fed hole.

Many times you find these saplings growing under a Neem tree. Just uproot one carefully, and plant it in a whole 12 to 20 inches deep. Water and allowed to grow.

You can also sprout them in a pot, if you want.

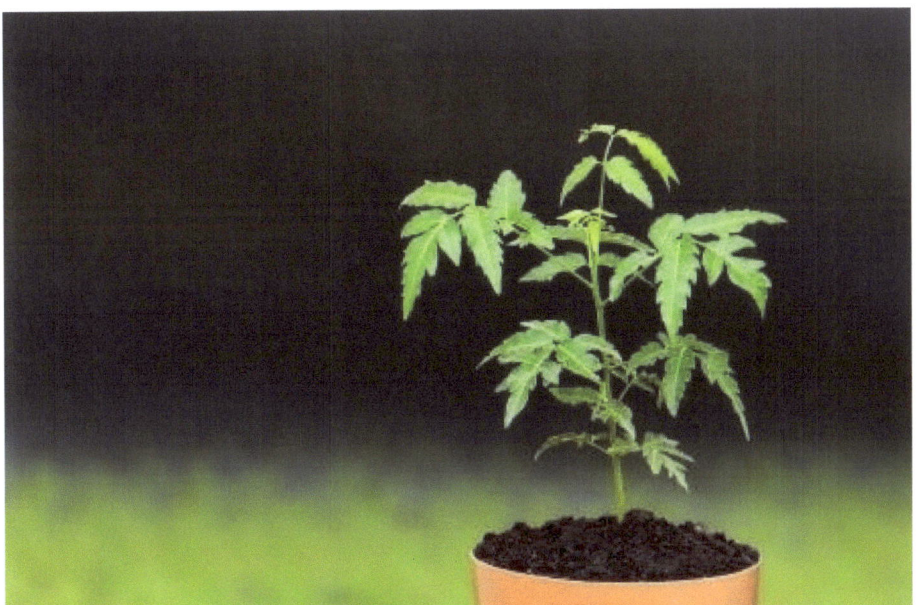

I know of a rooftop gardener who is going a Neem tree on the corner of her terrace in a water barrel. Of course, it is not a full-fledged tree, it is just a trunk with lots of branches, and it cannot expand. But it is growing and she uses the leaves boiled in water as a face wash. She also uses its twigs to brush her teeth. That shows that the will to survive in a Neem is great.

Here is another URL which you are going to find extremely useful and informative.

http://en.howtopedia.org/wiki/How_to_Grow_Neem_Trees

Neem in Ancient Medicine

The flowers and the leaves were used since ancient times to make herbal teas, which are considered to be the best remedy in which you can purify the blood. It is not only the Indians, who considered this as a blood purifier, the Persian ancient medical system also considered this to be an excellent medium to get rid of impurities in the blood.

When the Persian – or let us say the middle Asian – conquerors came to India in the 11th and 12th century, it is natural that they brought with them the knowledge of their medicines and their culture. Their doctors immediately set about utilizing the collected knowledge from the herbs, spices and trees indigenous to India. And that is why they began using Neem Leaves to prevent infections, brought about by wounds, and as a skin purifier.

Even today the cases of pimples, eczema and other skin diseases are very rare in places where there are plenty of Neem trees. You just go and pluck off some green and older leaves. Then you get someone in the kitchen to boil these leaves in water for you. The oldsters used to drink this decoction when they were young, but we are definitely not so stoic or brave. So, this water is going to be used as bathwater and external cleansing water until the skin reaches its natural glowing condition.

The Flowers of the Neem

Just imagine people living in unhygienic conditions in ancient times. They knew nothing about cleanliness and germs. So the moment somebody fell sick, they needed a natural remedy, which would heal. So imagine a child,

2000 years ago, playing about in the mud among livestock. Germs are abundant. He rubbed his eyes and soon finds his eyes getting infected.

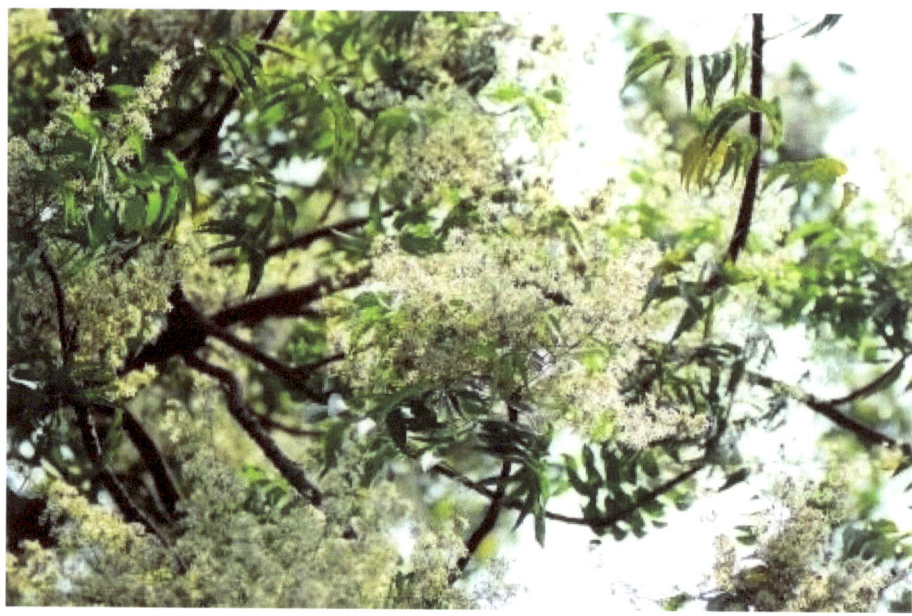

His mother is immediately going to boil flowers of the Neem and wash his eyes, three times a day with that water. She does not know that they are antiseptic. But she knows that they are going to prevent her son's eyes from worsening and he possibly going blind.

Traditional Kajal

Kajal is the black Kohl , which the Egyptians, the Persians, and the Indians used to wear since ancient times, to make their eyes look even more mysterious and mystical. Nowadays, you have this Kohl in expensive pencils produced by Lakme or L'Oreal.

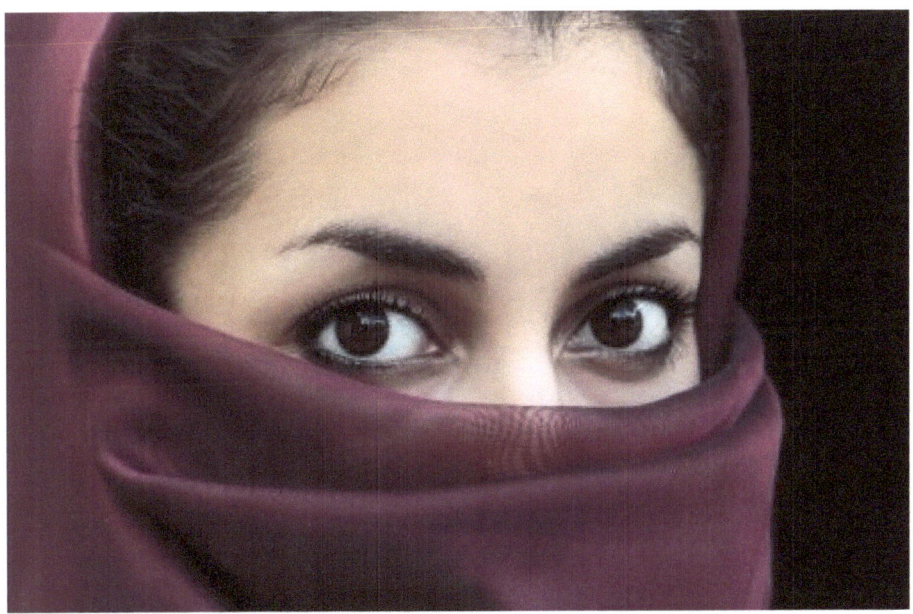

Kohl is a necessary part of every Oriental lovely's beauty arsenal.

This is the traditional way in which I saw Kohl being made, in the villages, as it had been done through centuries.

Take some fresh Neem flowers and wrap them up in a cotton swab. Make it into a lamp wick. Now put some Desi ghee in an earthenware lamp. Also add a little bit of Neem bark and a powdered almond to the ghee in the lamp. Light the lamp. [You are going to get to know how to make Desi ghee in the appendix. This is the Indian clarified butter, and is used as an antiseptic to heal as well as a healthy natural food to keep you fit and fine and long-lived.]

Now place this lit lamp between two bricks and invert a metal tray. Let the soot collect on the surface of the metal. This is your original kohl. You are going to mix it with just that much of powdered alum, which covers the surface of a pinhead. .97 g! Add 20 g or two large teaspoonfuls of desi ghee to make up an oily sooty paste called Kajra or kajal .

This was collected in ancient times in a copper container, with an applier. In Persia, this was called *Soorma*- just the soot ash. I still have my great-grandmother's *soormchi* made of copper. People had them made of silver too in ancient times. Though of course, the soorma in it has gone the way of all herbal creations.

How to Apply Kajal?

Just outline your eyes with the applier, on which surface this paste has adhered. It is definitely not going to hurt your eyes. You may find your eyes watering a bit, but that is because it has come in contact with the cold metal. The tears are also going to wash away the excess Kohl, but still leave enough behind to keep your eyes looking dark, beautiful, Mystic, healthy and mysterious!

If you have collected this in a little box, do not worry, you can use a small Neem twig as an applier!

That is what is done by people who could not be bothered about soormchis in gold, silver, or copper.

Curing Eye Infections

I saw this procedure being practiced by a grandmother whose child had some eye problems. Naturally, not being near a Doctor, she used this ancient remedy to get rid of dimming of vision, eye infections, eye irritations, and other eye related ailments.

She dried some Neem leaves in the shade, and then put them in a clay pot, 30 minutes on the fire, and they were burnt to a crisp. This ash was then collected and then ground with lemon juice. This leafy ash powder was then collected and used as a kajal twice a day until the eyes were cured. And they were cured. No irritations, no infections, and the vision improved drastically.

Scientific research, anyone? Easy, lemon, and Neem are both antiseptic.

Neem Seeds as a Pesticide

Since ancient times, Neem seeds have been used as a pesticide, as well as an organic fertilizer. 800 g of Neem extract/oil from the seeds, can preserve hundred kilograms of stored grain from fungus and other pests. You can also sprinkle plenty of dried Neem leaves in your storage barn and on the storage sacks, and prevent pest attacks.

Neem Seeds as a Paralysis/Stroke Massage Oil

Neem oil has been in use to massage the affected areas during paralysis or strokes because it is as powerful as mustard oil. This is considered to be a very good medium to increase the circulatory system in your muscles and revive dead tissue.

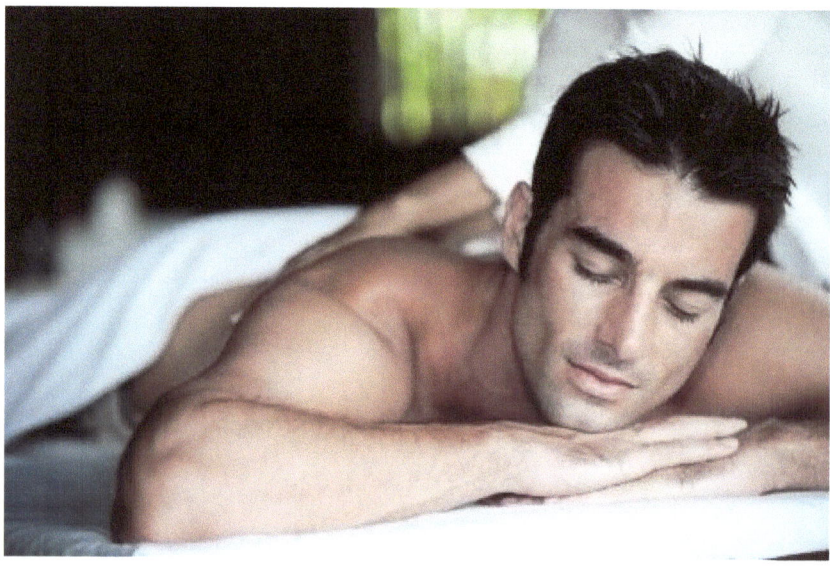

An occasional massage is good for your health. It is also good when you are sick.

Also, if you feel a loss of sensation in your hands or in your feet, due to any reason, including the cold, massage that area with Neem oil. That is going to get your system up and about again.

Curing Piles

Suffering from hemorrhoids? You may want to apply my Neem ointment given below to the affected area in order to get relief from pain and to heal. Also take out 2 tablespoons full of ripe Neem fruit pulp and stir them in water.

Gulp down twice a day. You are going to find your system getting cured from inside. This is considered to be a time tested remedy. No operations, no drugs, no more pain.

You can also cured piles by making up a mixture of one peppercorn and 20 g of powdered Neem seeds. Mix them together and make pills the size of lemon drops or small marbles. Swallow one pill with water twice a day.

You could also apply a paste of the seeds ground with water with a cotton wad on the affected area. But I would suggest the Neem ointment!

Sweet Neem?

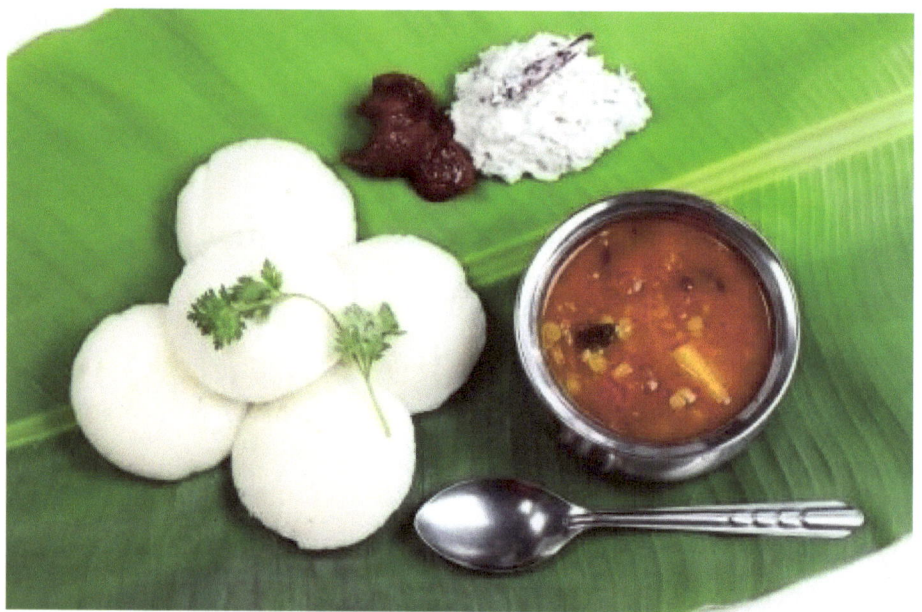

This traditional South Indian breakfast of idli, sambhar and coconut chutney is well garnished with curry leaves in the rasam and sambhar. It is served on a banana leaf.

Yes, there is a variety of Neem, which is definitely not bitter. You know this plant as the Curry leaf tree. If you have eaten any authentic South Indian dishes, these leaves add delicious taste and distinction to the sambhars and rasams. In fact, I have one of them growing in my balcony in a pot. So whenever I want to spice up anything, including meat dishes, I just add a couple of freshly washed leaves.

Halitosis

Do I suffer from bad breath? Or is it just something I ate?

Sweet Neem, just like the Neem, an excellent method to get rid of mouth odor. There was a time when I used to suffer from halitosis brought about by a lot – of – meat – diet. Naturally, I was asked by my grandmother to chew those bitter Neem leaves, before I left for the office.

So there I was, chewing the cud and making faces like any bovine, swishing that terribly bitter mouthful around my mouth, and then spitting it out at the nearest rosebush after five minutes, followed with gagging noises to the tune of *eyakkargghptchaaa*....

The taste was removed by rinsing out my mouth with a glass full of salty water.

Any sort of mouth infection does not have a chance with such a drastic treatment. Within five days, I had found myself rid of toothache and halitosis. And at that time, alas, I did not know that the Sweet Neem was equally effective. But this I know. No mouthwashes, ever!

Before I go out, I just have to chew for five minutes on Sweet Neem leaves – without any accompanying noises and faces – and my breath is going to smell as fresh as Neem!

You may also want to try brushing your teeth with Neem twigs. This is a story told to me by my uncle, who was an experienced commando Army officer. Well, he was in terrorist zone under continuous attack, and how did they get to know all about the presence of those wily foxes, the Commandos?

That was because the commandos brushed their teeth with chalky and scented mouth freshening toothpaste, and spat out the foam near any water source. Those terrorists being more of the land, definitely did not use such modern teeth cleansing materials. If they ever brushed their teeth, they always used twigs, as their ancestors had done.

So after that, uncle got his men to brush their teeth with salt and water, or with Neem twigs, if available in the vicinity. He also made sure that soap was made taboo in any commando pack. If they wanted to have a bath, they would be better off using riverbed mud to scrub off the dirt and the grime.

This may not look very sophisticated to a cultured mind, but this is the best way in which you can keep your teeth clean, your gums healthy and prevent to diseases.

Neem Seeds as Poultry and Cattle Feed

Believe it or not, the remnants remaining after the oil has been extracted from the seeds are excellent as poultry and cattle feed. You may also want to husk the seeds, and remove the pulp. The seeds can then be powdered and mixed with your poultry feed. It has been proved that this increases the yield of eggs and their quality.

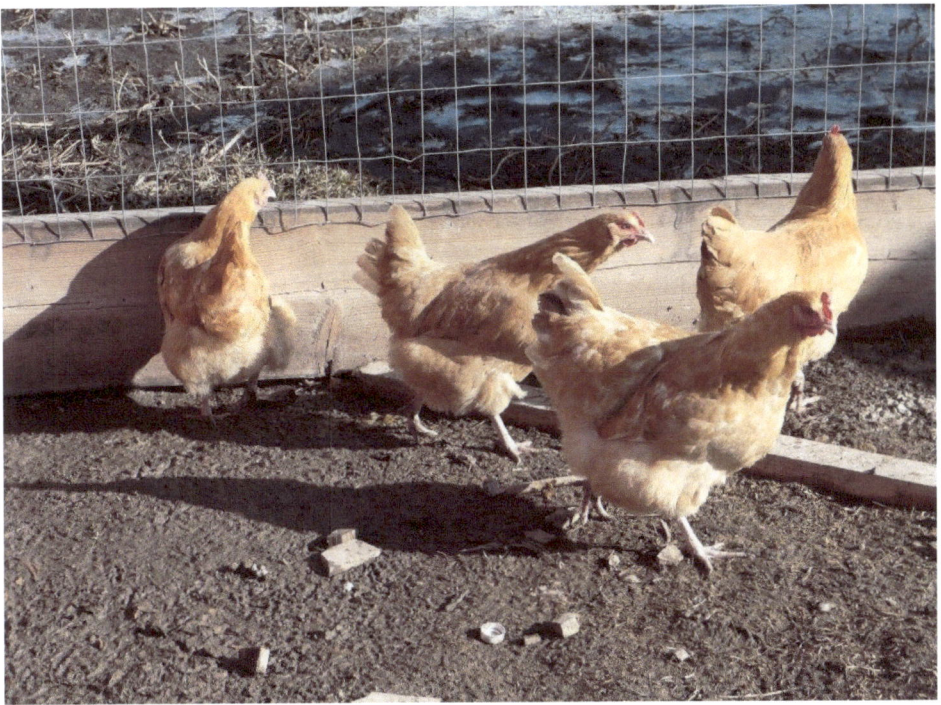

Try feeding your chicks on organic feed like Neem seeds, chopped greens, and dry fish meal.

Preserving Clothes and Books

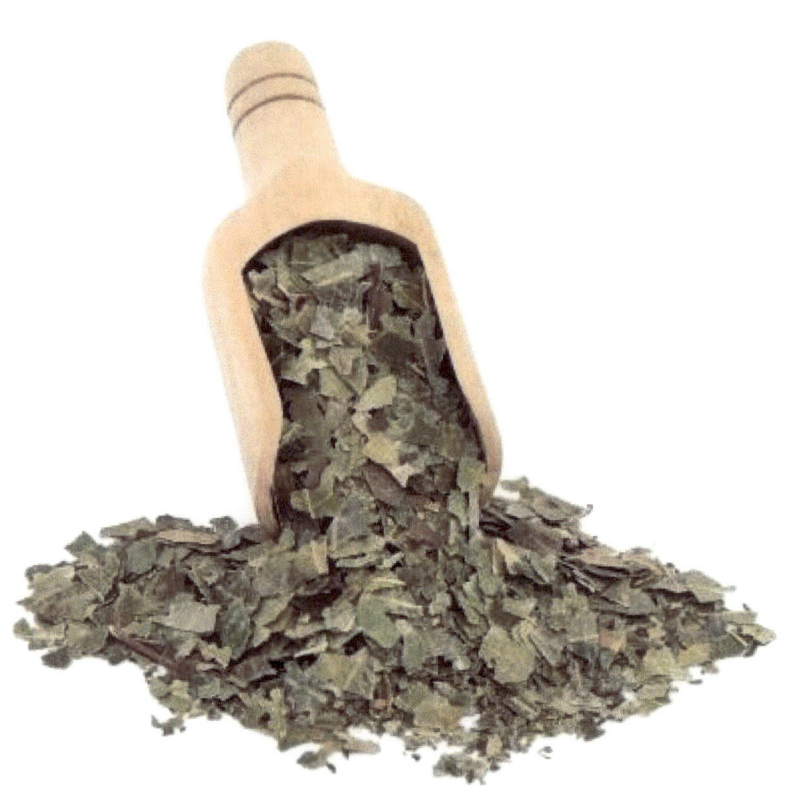

Dried powdered leaves of the Neem

This is what I learned from elders who do not bother about naphthalene balls to protect their precious woolens. That is because they have Neem leaves ready at hand. The next time you are storing away woolens or even your precious expensive clothes, do not put in naphthalene balls, because that is going to leave a characteristic odor, when you take out those clothes next winter.

Dry 15 to 20 fresh Neem leaves in the shade. I normally dry them in more quantities, because I preserve my books with these dry leaves too. That means that I do not have to worry about moths and silverfish biting my precious books.

The best thing about dry leaves of Neem is that, when you take out your clothes next winter, they are going to smell fresh, instead of smelling moldy or smelling of damp. Do not dry them directly in the sun. That is going to get rid of all the essential oils is necessary to keep all these pests away.

So look for a shady portion in your sunny balcony, spread out a cloth and put all these leaves on the cloth. Fold the cloth and leave for four – five days. You are going to have powdery Neem leaves.

Now once you have them, put your favorite clothes on a piece of cloth. Spread the cloth, and then spread a layer of powdered Neem leaves. Then place another suit – woolen jacket – any expensive dress – on top of this layer and spread another layer of leaves.

So you have a sandwich of clothes and Neem leaves. Wrap up the bundle and store away.

I used to get very annoyed when I used to see these powdered leaves littering the ground, when I took out my woollies lovingly put in store by my grandmother. There is an easy solution for that. You can make small cloth pouches with squares of cotton cloth, with the leaves in them, and knotted up. These are going to be placed in judicial positions all over your clothes bundles and in your wardrobe. For individual dress packing, place one pouch under the dress and one over it.

You can even place them in the pockets of your coats, blazers and jackets.

I normally place these pouches in the bookshelves of my library. I have never suffered from silverfish eating my books and making me groan with dismay when I open them up years later.

Curing Wounds with Neem

Remember that no wound is going to get cured, if it is not well cleaned beforehand. So it should be washed with Neem water to get rid of any foreign materials present in that wound. It is also going to prevent germ infection in the initial stages.

Infections occur only when wounds have been allowed to fester without anybody taking care of them. There was a time when honey was used to cure infections. But that was only when you do not have Neem around.

Cleaning Infections

Cleaning of the infection can be done in these ways –

Take some boiling water in a glass bowl. Now add some Neem leaves to this water. Infuse for 15 minutes, so that the essential oils of the Neem can be soaked up in the water.

I normally add Neem oil, if I do not have Neem leaves. I also prefer boiling the water with the Neem leaves. Any method is going to do, you are getting an infusion, are not you.

Just dip some cotton in this liquid, and wash the wounded area 8-9 times. You may also want to cool this boiled water, and irrigate that area in a stream of antiseptic. Then bandage with a cotton cloth and allow the water to dry. Then lift up the cloth and apply the Neem ointment. Then bandage and allow to heal. Do this every day, and as often as required, until the wound has healed properly and all the infection has disappeared.

In India, the British used to make up a mixture of potassium permanganate and Neem Leaves in water to wash any cuts, bruises and wounds. This is an extremely sensible measure, because after all potassium permanganate was also used to disinfect fruit and vegetables before cooking.

The pink water was called pinky- paani by the British Memsahibs . So one could imagine them yelling at the cooks, if pinky paani was used to wash the fruit and vegetables or not.

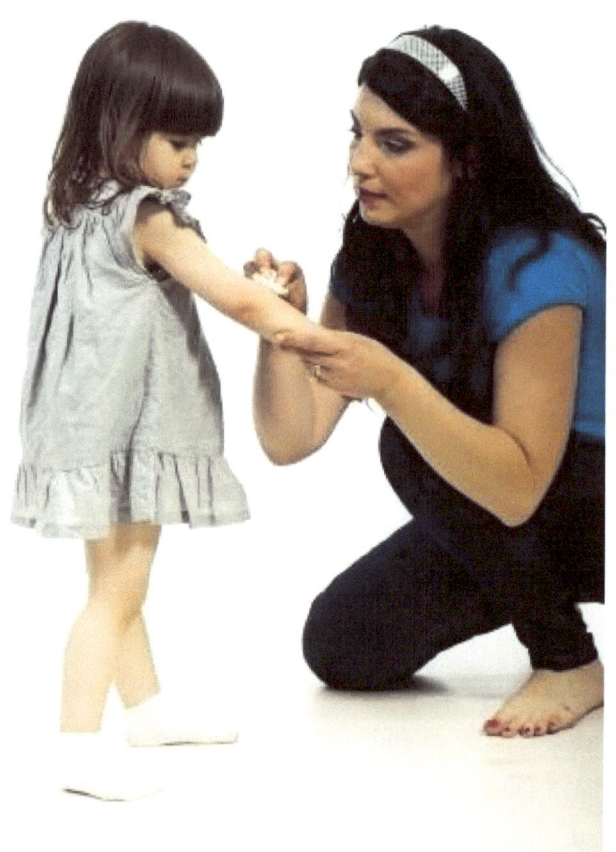

Making a Neem Poultice

If you have not had an opportunity to make an appointment, or it is not ready at hand, you can bandage the wounds with a Neem poultice. This is done by crushing fresh Neem leaves and applying them on the wound. Cover up with a cloth and bandage. This is going to prevent any further infection.

My Own Neem Ointment

Before I give you my recipe for a Neem ointment, I am going to tell you all about how you are going to infuse Neem oil, which is going to be used in balms, salves and ointments.

A salve is the oil thickened with beeswax, melted together in the ratio of 4:1

.

An ointment has the ratio of 10 to 1. 10 parts oil to one part wax.

If you have the time and the inclination, and there is lots of sun outside, you may want to infuse the oils in the sun.

The Slow Sun Method

I normally choose a light vegetable oil like sunflower oil, but my grandmother used to infuse herbs in desi ghee (Clarified butter) or freshly homemade butter.

I have noticed that the desi ghee infusions are more powerful, because of their concentrated power to heal. But then everybody knows my tight pockets would scream blue murder if I spent lots of money on pure and expensive desi ghee, just for the sole purpose of using it in infusions instead of eating it and so gaining full value for my money, so if you do have a good supply of homemade desi ghee , be my guest and use it !

By the way somehow, everybody in India and around it knows that desi ghee is the best agent for painless healing of cuts and wounds.

Anyway, collect your Neem leaves and Neem fruit. Then, fill a large glass jar (we call it a *achaar wala martban* or pickle jar bottle) with a good vegetable oil, or homemade butter or ghee. This glass jar normally comes in sizes of two – 5 L capacity! But you do not have to fill it up to the brim with ghee!

Add the Neem leaves until they are covered with the oil but are not tightly packed, (I found out that 10 to 12 handfuls of the leaves did me just fine, there was enough of space for all of them to breathe.)

Cover with an air tight lid and leave in direct sunshine. The leaves will turn brown after a couple of days. Remove them and add fresh leaves. Repeat this procedure until the oil is tinged green. (The more changes you do, the more Neem extract you are going to have in the oil in your precious bottle.)

People living in tropical regions are very lucky because we have a good supply of rose flowers as well as direct sunlight, but in many Western countries it is tough luck when all ye sun deprived people have to go up to 20 or more changes because of the uncertain summer season and rainy weather. The more you persevere, and the more patient you are, the more this rather long method captures the natural power of this wonderful curative.

When you find the oil has turned really green, you would like to make some natural salves from them.

Another Neem Oil Method

Take three fistfuls of fresh green leaves and add them to 250 g of boiling hot oil. Allow to cook until all the leaves are burnt. Now this very powerful oil needs to be filtered, and placed in a glass bottle. This is an excellent remedy to apply on Burns and wounds, if you do not want to turn it into an ointment.

Here is my Neem ointment.

- ☐ **2/3 cups cooking oil,**
- ☐ **15 g beeswax, grated or chopped into small pieces,**
- ☐ **50 g infused oil**

Put the oils, and beeswax into a small pan. Put the lid on and stand it into the large water pan. Carefully pour water into the larger water pan. Here you have to be careful that the level of the water is lower than that of the level of the oil, because this oil container is not going to have a lid upon it. Keep stirring until the wax is melted.

Allow to cool a little, take out the inner pan and remove the lid. Put this ointment in a handy container and use it to heal wounds. Naturally, these ointments keep for many months.

You may ask me if I have tried making ointments out of Neem oil, so plentiful in the East. The answer is yes, and it works equally well. But I use only about 25 g of Neem oil, because it is very powerful and very concentrated.

Neem Burn Remedy

The ointment recipe I gave to you above is for wound infection prevention, but this is an effective remedy to prevent burns from getting infected .

Add 250 g of Neem oil to 125 g of wax. Now add 1 kg of fresh green Neem leaves juice, 50 g of powdered Neem root bark and 25 g of dried Neem leaf ash. I do not think I have left anything out in this very powerful concoction!

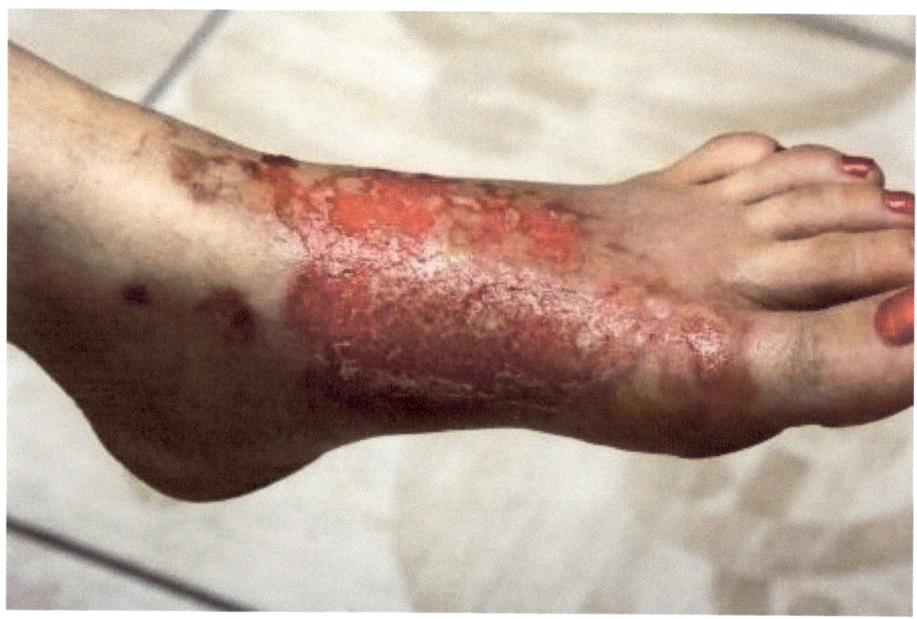

Now, heat the oil with the liquid on slow heat until the oil is reduced to half its quantity. Now add the wax. Then both of them have turned into us. Most mixture, you are going to add the Neem root powder and the ash. Just heat for another one minute and cool. This is the best remedy in which you can cure bun infections. Try it out right now.

In fact, I have this in my kitchen, because that is the place where I get burnt through oil splats and by accidentally touching red-hot utensils.

Also, when the burns are healed, I get rid of the scars, by a mixture of turmeric paste with honey. So no one can say that hey, that burn scar looks so… so… *[Embarrassed muttering fading away, unless the person is really insensitive.]*

Sprains

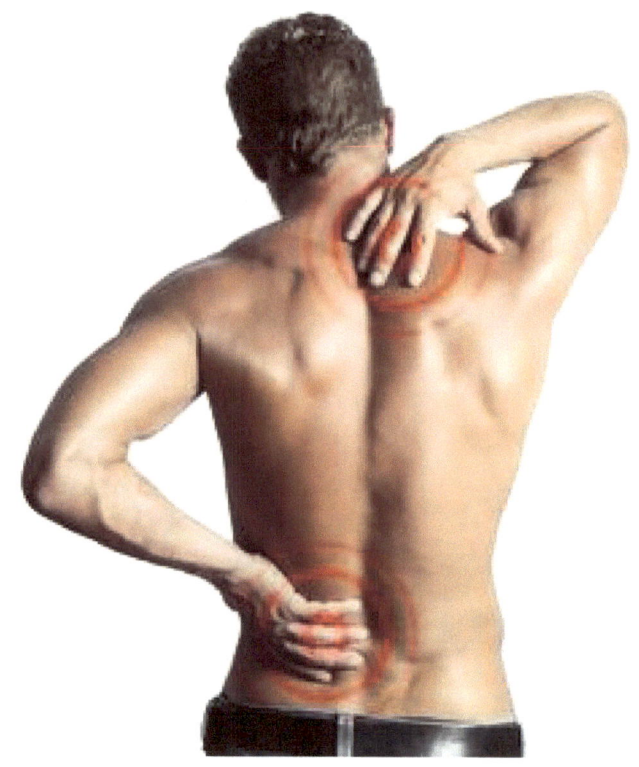

If you find yourself suffering from sprains, especially when the tissue has swollen up and you find it very painful to move, try this remedy. Just heat some fresh Neem leaves in mustard oil. Then add some turmeric to this mixture, and apply, when still hot to the affected area and bandage tight. This is definitely going to have a beneficial visible effect on the sprain.

Well, I know that it is the turmeric, which heals the sprain. The Neem cools that inflamed area down and the mustard oil is the medium, which heals and cures.

Prickly Heat

This is such an amazing remedy to get rid of prickly heat, especially in the summer, that I wonder why people do not use it more. They would rather sprinkle themselves with prickly heat powder with salicyclic acid and they are perfectly satisfied with the temporary relief, they get with this powder. But try this idea. The moment summer starts coming in, and you know that you are going to suffer from prickly heat, just add seven drops of Neem oil in a bucket full of water.

If you want to soak in the bath, you can add 2 tablespoons of Neem oil, because of the larger quantity of water. Then scrub your skin thoroughly with this antiseptic powerful bathing medium. No prickly heat ever.

So, okay, you want to know about what about the people who prefer showers to bathtubs or buckets? Easy, put three drops of Neem oil in a mug full of water. Just dip your sponge in it, and apply it all over your body. Do that 3 – 4 times before you shower. After you have showered, repeat the sponging two more times. No skin infection, this summer, or any other summer.

Pain in Joints

If you are suffering from joint pain, you can cure this ailment by making a paste of water and the inner portion of the Neem bark. Apply this on the ailing area three times a day. You are going to see a positive effect within the week.

Do your Shoes Bite?

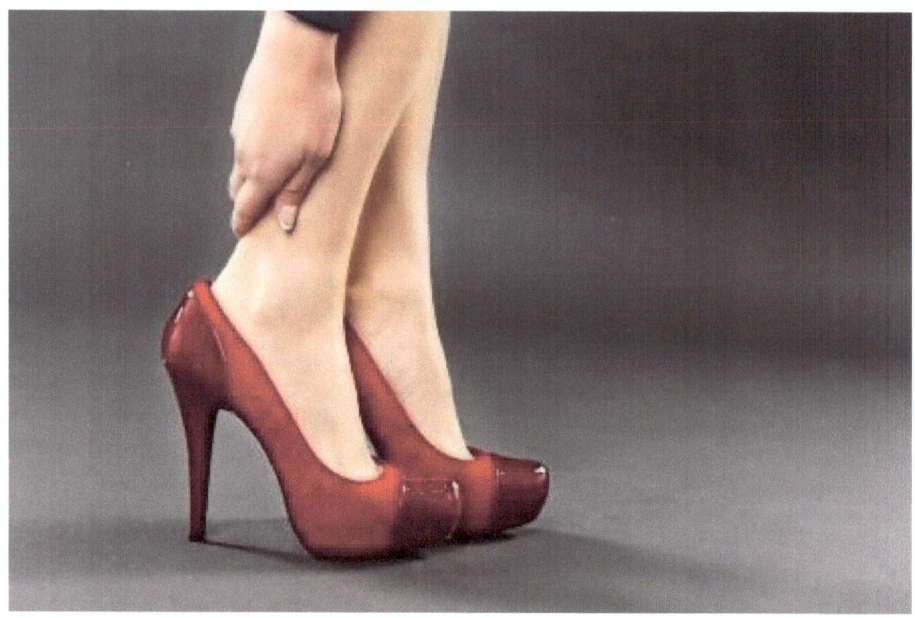

Ill fitting shoes? Potential foot trouble!

Believe it or not, one has suffered. After all, there was that mouthwatering display of well -designed shoes at a really reasonable rate. I defy anybody not to get tempted. I am not Imelda Marcos with hundred pairs of shoes, but the ones I have need to fit me well. Unfortunately, sometimes they fit me excellently when I am trying them on, in the shop. But by the time I come back home, my feet are killing me literally and figuratively.

This is normally what happens when the shoe pinches. Also, you may find your skin getting so chafed that it might get infected. You may never be able to wear those shoes again, because you remember the pain associated with them. That is when your heels, your toes and your feet may find them raw and chafed.

So all you have to do is cure these chafes by mixing some Neem oil in wax, and applying all over the affected areas.

I would suggest that you put off leaving wearing those shoes until your feet are healed.

But if you have to wear them, protect your skin by making up a mixture of Neem leaf Ash in Neem oil, and then applying all over your feet, putting on your socks and then putting on the shoes.

Another remedy is you can massage your feet with Neem oil, and then sprinkle Neem ash all over your feet. So any chances of any potential wounds can immediately be tackled by the Neem already present on your epidermis.

How to Make Neem Ash?

Just get together some fresh Neem leaves and a clay pot. Put the leaves in the pot and place on heat. They are going to be burned to an ash. This ash can be collected and put in a bottle, to be used whenever needed, especially when you do not have fresh Neem leaves around.

Leukoderma Cure

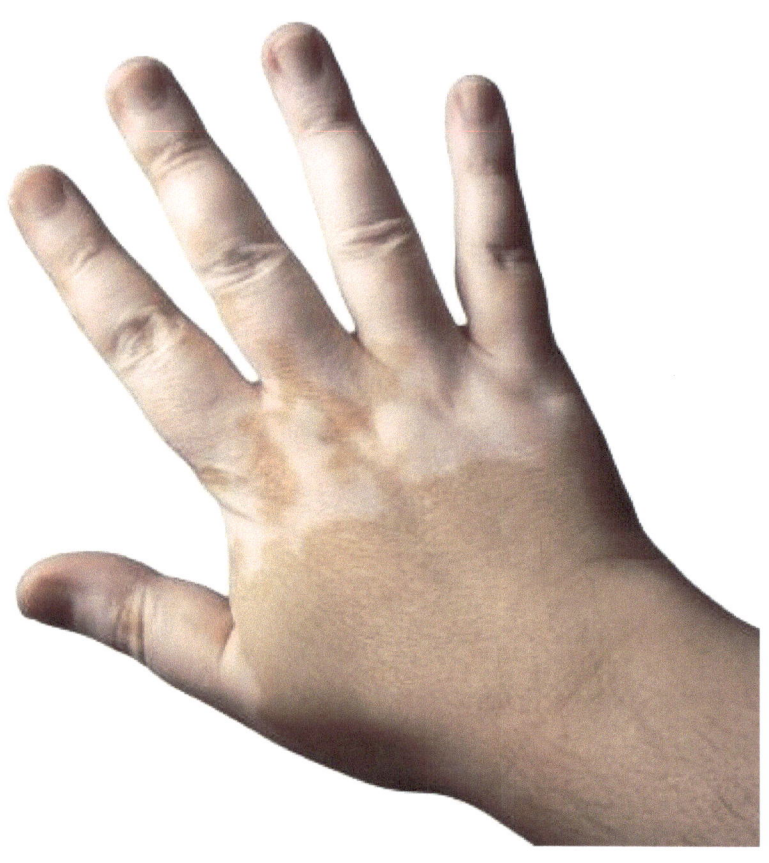

Make a dried leaf Ash of Neem leaves and using it mixed with Desi ghee in a paste. Apply it all over the white patches. You may find a visible effect on the skin, because that gets the skin melanin growing again, unless you are genetically prone to no melanin in the body.

Fever Cure

Do you know that Neem bark was used to cure periodic fever and even malaria, when cinchona was not around. This was discovered by Dr. D. D. White in 1803. He made a concoction of Neem bark and fed it to patients suffering from periodic fever. And they were cured.

But then Neem bark boiled in water has been used as a remedy to get rid of fever down the ages. You may try it, if you are feeling feverish and do not want to go to the doctor. The bark is bitter, just like cinchona.

The internal part of the bark is used for curing malaria. In ancient times, if a person suffered from ordinary fever, the family members would just collect the new and green stalks of Neem leaves. They would then grind them up with water and feed that liquid to the patient until the fever was cured.

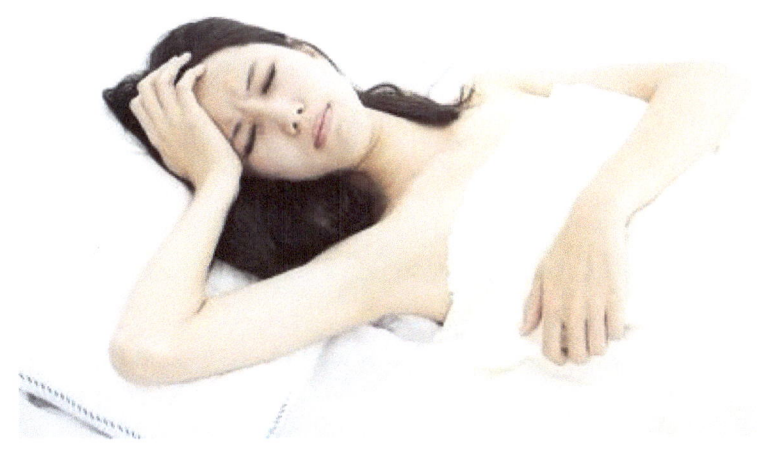

Getting Rid of Bedbugs

This is an extremely good and useful remedy for all those people who find themselves in bedbug infested areas. These include hotels, and other residential places all over the world. So the next time you smell that sickly sweet smell, which tells you that there are bedbugs around, do not go destroying all your bedding. Instead, fumigate the bedding, and all the furniture in the area with a mixture of sulfur and Neem leaves. Put them in a container and light the mixture.

Shut the door and the windows while this mixture is smoking in that affected area. Open it, after two hours. No bedbugs. Even better, no other pests like cockroaches and ants. They disappear, or just suffocate and die.

Malarial Fumigation

Also, this is the best way to get rid of mosquitoes, especially when there is a chance of a malarial or a dengue epidemic. Take a bunch of Neem leaves, make them into a torch and go around the place, allowing the Neem smoke to fill the area. You can call this natural Neem fumigation.

I suggested this natural remedy to the town's municipality, instead of their very powerful and poisonous potential harmful fumigatory sprayed pesticide, – which leaves eyes burning, and asthmatic patients miserable – but the look on their faces was about as bland and blank as a solid and immovable brick wall. This idea and initiative will not assimilate in these hidebound mental limits.

How to Make Neem Soap

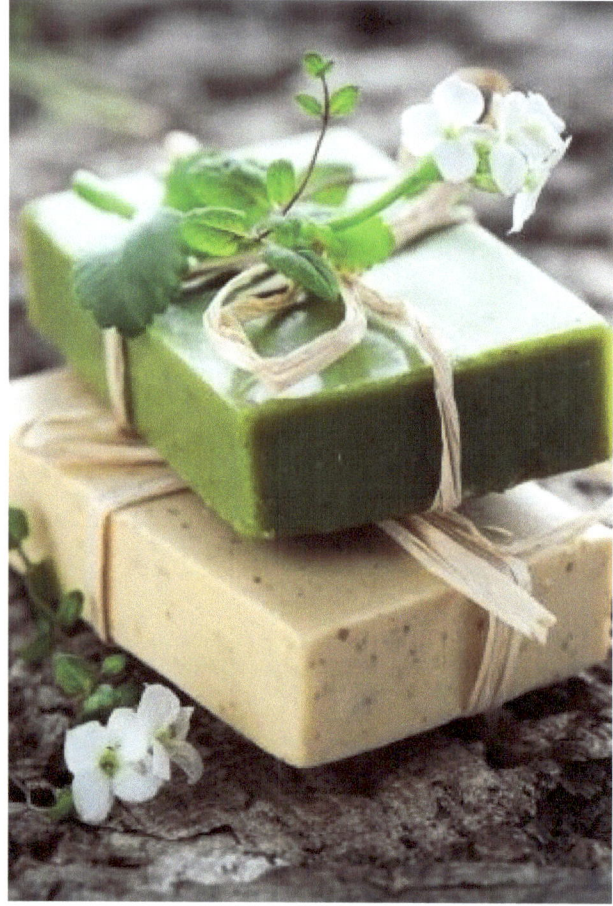

Soaps you make yourself with natural essential oils are much better and healthier for you in the long run.

If you go into any natural resources/products shop in the East, and asked them for Neem soap, they are going to give you a soap under the brand name of Margosa. It is extremely popular, and of course it is extremely effective.

So make your own Margosa at home. Now remember, that every soap, which you get in the market has caustic soda in it, so I do not want to use any item which can burn my hands or harm me. I know plenty of people, who make washing soap, right at home, but they do not mind a little bit of caustic soda acting caustically on their skins.

So I am giving you an extremely easy recipe with which you can make Neem soap right at home.

Just go to your craft shop and ask for glycerin-based soap base, which can be melted and poured. This is extremely mild. Now the amount of Neem oil that you are going to put in it, is going to depend on whether you want the soap to be oily, are you just wanted to be dry.

If you want really powerful Neem soap to keep your head and scalp healthy, especially when you are using it as a shampoo instead of chemical-based shampoos, or to cure parasite infections, make sure the amount of Neem is 20% of the original quantity of soap base.

Just cut the soap base into manageable chunks. Put it in a double boiler for melting. If you are making 250 g of soap, 5% of the oil is going to be about 13 to 15 g of Neem oil. Make it 2 tablespoons. That is more than enough.

Melt the soap in the double boiler. You can also do that in the microwave, but remember to stir occasionally, if you are using this particular melting process.

Once the soap has melted, just stir in the oil, and there you are, you are done, you just need to pour it into molds to set. You may also want to add in some essential oils, but in the East, one prefers to smell pure Neem. He is reassured that he is bathing with the real thing, the best skin cure and the best hair and scalp cleanser.

Also, make sure that the original soap base, if you cannot get glycerin is made up of saponified and natural oils. Do not buy chemical-based soap bases.

Appendix

How to Make Desi Ghee

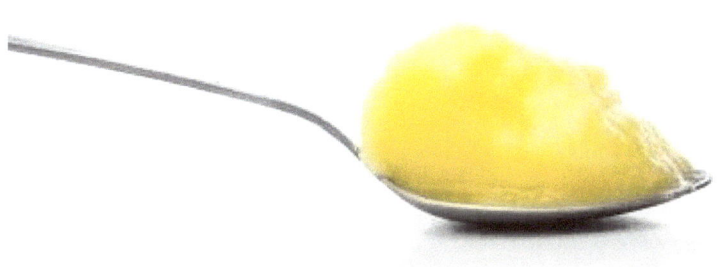

Desi ghee is clarified butter, grainy in consistency and golden yellow in color. It is extremely concentrated and is a very powerful healing agent. It is normally used in the making up of herbal medicines, because it is made of pure creamy milk butter. It is also used in making beauty creams, potions, lotions and other skin ointments.

It has a powerful aroma, and that is why only just a spoonful is added to fry meats. It is going to float on the surface of the meat dish, after it has been cooked, so you need to stir the gravy before serving. Also, the food is not going to taste greasy, even though it looks like it has been swimming in fat.

Desi ghee is the concentrated form of pure butter, which is heated to reduce the butter of all the impurities as well as moisture. This concentrated butter is normally used in Eastern cuisine, for searing meat, sautéing and frying food, because they offer its higher burning point. You make this at home by taking 2 pounds of best unsalted butter and melting it in a heavy bottomed pan. Allow the butter to liquefy on low heat for about 40 minutes. Maintain this simmering point, until all of the moisture in the butter has evaporated. The impurities are going to sink to the bottom of the pan. Remember to keep stirring the butter, so that it does not burn.

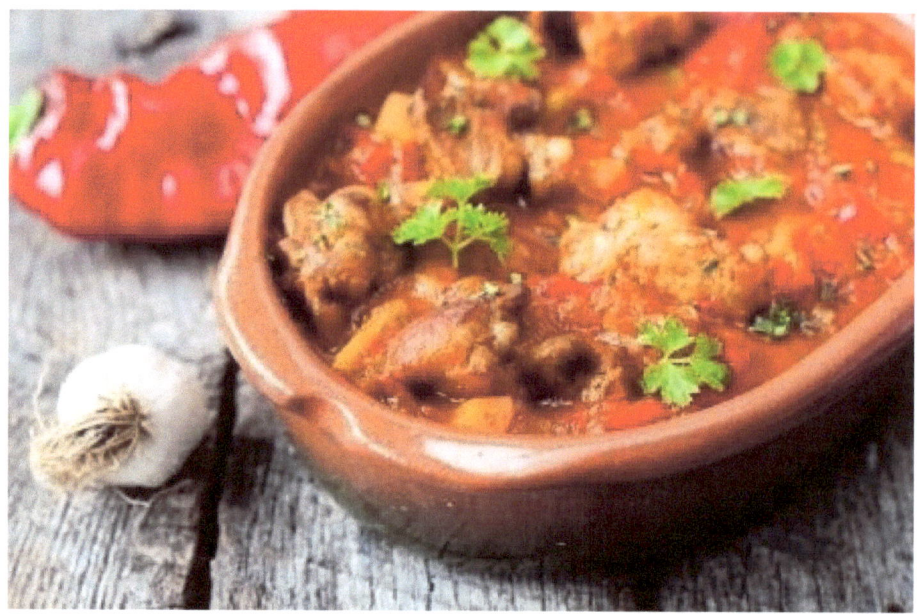

Yes, that is Desi Ghee floating on the surface. That is why the cook needs to give this a stir, before she serves it up to an appreciative, and hungry audience. This does not leave the food greasy, however oily it may look.

Pour off the clear butter and strain it through several thicknesses of muslin cloth. This butter is going to last for about a year, if it is placed in a cool and dry place. This butter is exorbitantly expensive. So in the East, people with easy access to plenty fresh milk make it right in their kitchens for crisp delicious frying results, and adding that taste of pure butter to all their dishes.

Conclusion

I hope you enjoyed this informative book on the magic of Neem. The Margot plant is one of the boons of nature to humankind. Each part of it is useful. I could have given you some recipes made up of Neem flowers, and eaten traditionally, but I have not tried them out, so I could not tell you how they taste.

Nevertheless, Neem flowers and fresh leaves is an integral part of cuisine in many parts of the East, in the form of lunch dishes, and chutneys.

Also, the ripe Neem fruit is edible, though, I have not seen anybody human eating the pulp. What a waste by not eating something, which cures!

So live happy, grow a Neem in your locality, allow it to flourish, and see how the breeze around it is purified. Believe it or not, Neem is considered to be the best air purifier, and there are plenty of cities in the West, which have decided to lower the pollution content in their areas by planting the Neem.

The Neem tree purifies the air for more than 50 feet around it. That is why people do not mind resting under a Neem, whenever they can, especially on hot summer days, even when traditionally the belief is prevalent that you should not sleep under a tree in the afternoon.

So now that you know all about the health giving benefits of the Neem, enjoy a happy and healthy life, appreciating the bounty of nature and all its goodies just for you.

Author Bio

Dueep Jyot Singh is a Management and IT Professional who managed to gather Postgraduate qualifications in Management and English and Degrees in Science, French and Education while pursuing different enjoyable career options like being an hospital administrator, IT,SEO and HRD Database Manager/ trainer, movie scriptwriter, theatre artiste and public speaker, lecturer in French, Marketing and Advertising, ex-Editor of Hearts On Fire (now known as Solsctice) Books Missouri USA, advice columnist and cartoonist, publisher and Aviation School trainer, ex- moderator on Medico.in, banker, student councilor ,travelogue writer … among other things! One fine morning, she decided that she had enough of killing herself by Degrees and went back to her first love -- writing. It's more enjoyable! She already has 48 published academic and 14 fiction- in- different- genre books under her belt.

When she is not designing websites or making Graphic design illustrations for clients , she is browsing through old bookshops hunting for treasures, of which she has an enviable collection – including R.L. Stevenson, O.Henry, Dornford Yates, Maurice Walsh, C.N.Williamson, Sapper, Bartimeus and the crown of her collection- Dickens "The Old Curiosity Shop," and so on… Just call her "Renaissance Woman" - collecting herbal remedies, acting like Universal Helping Hand/Agony Aunt, or escaping to her dear mountains for a bit of exploring, collecting herbs and plants, and trekking.

Check out some of the other Health Learning Series books at Amazon.com

Health Learning Series on Amazon

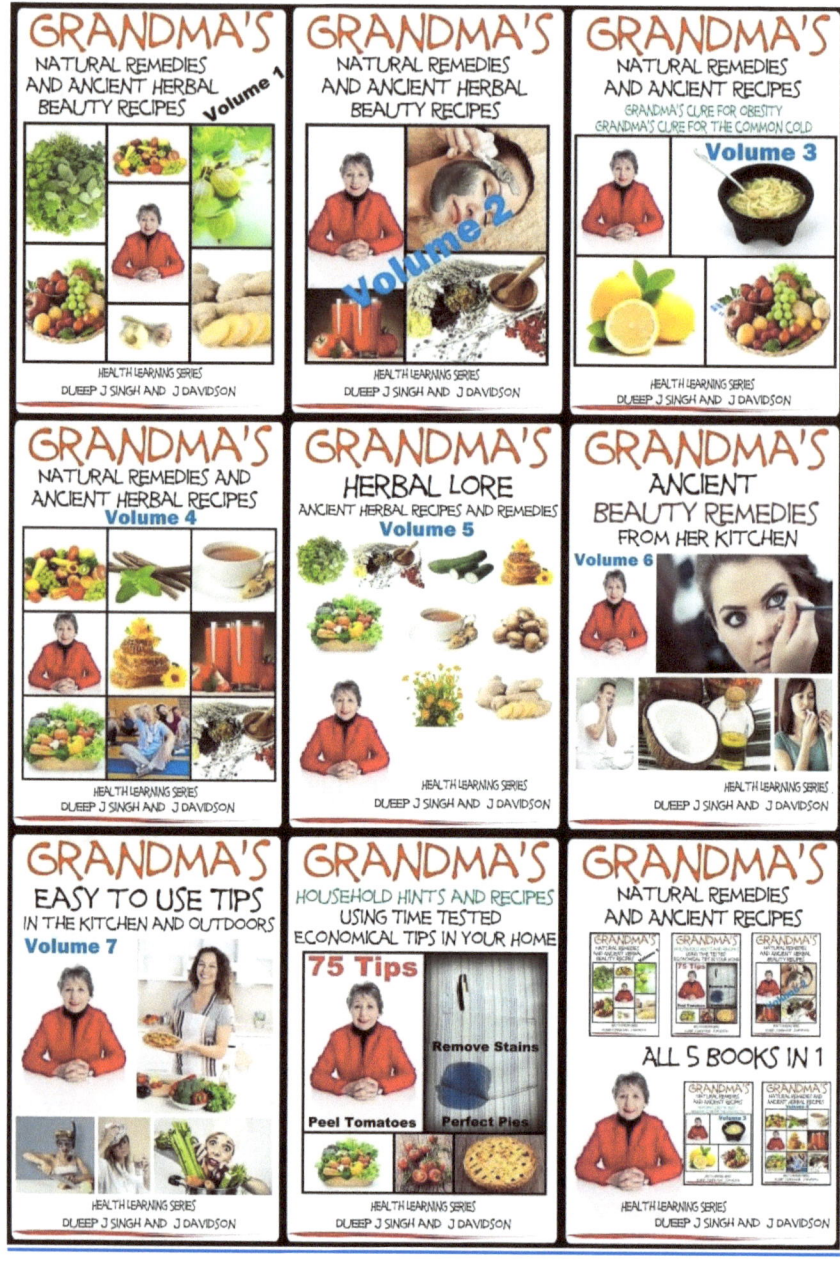

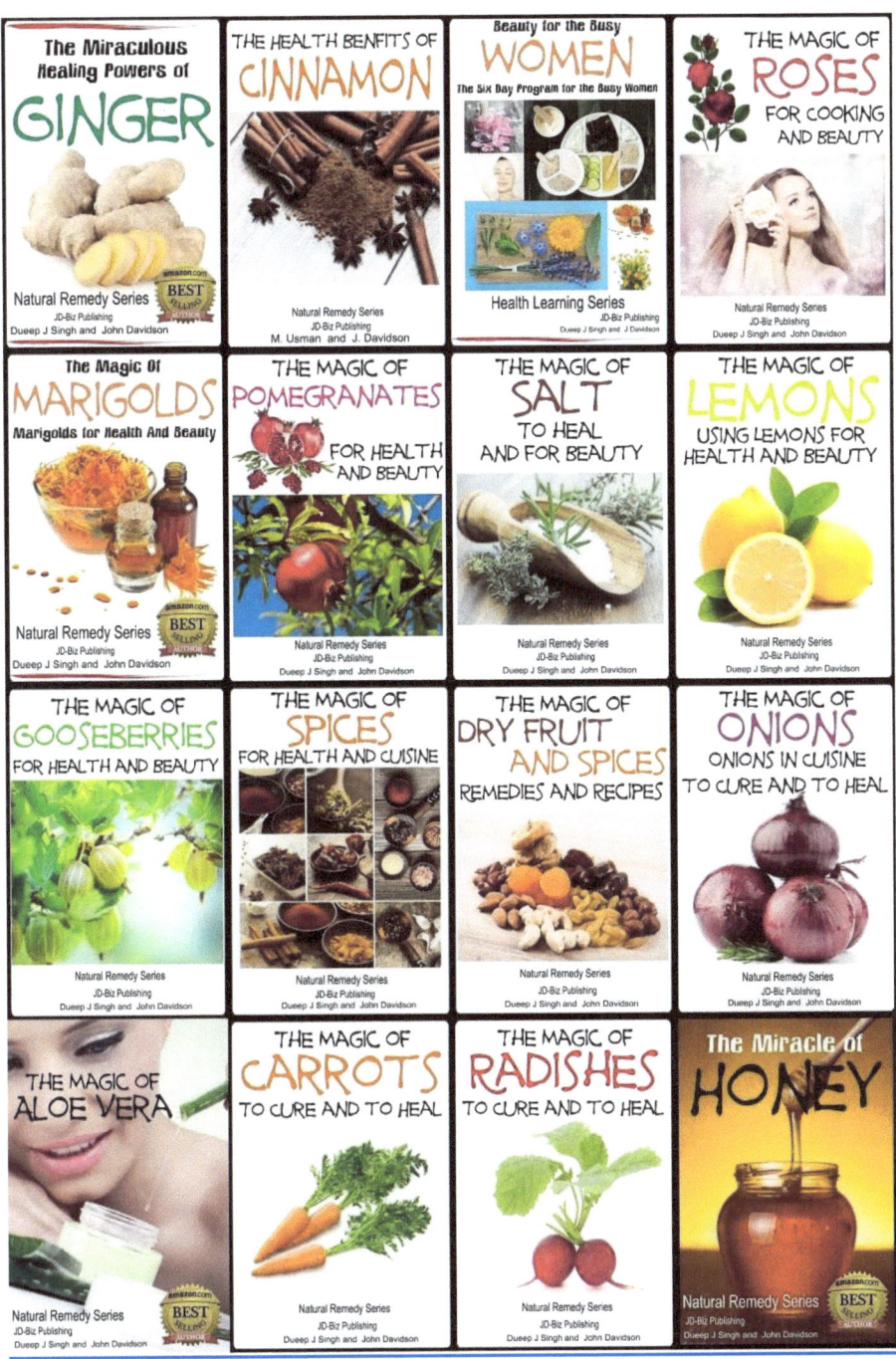

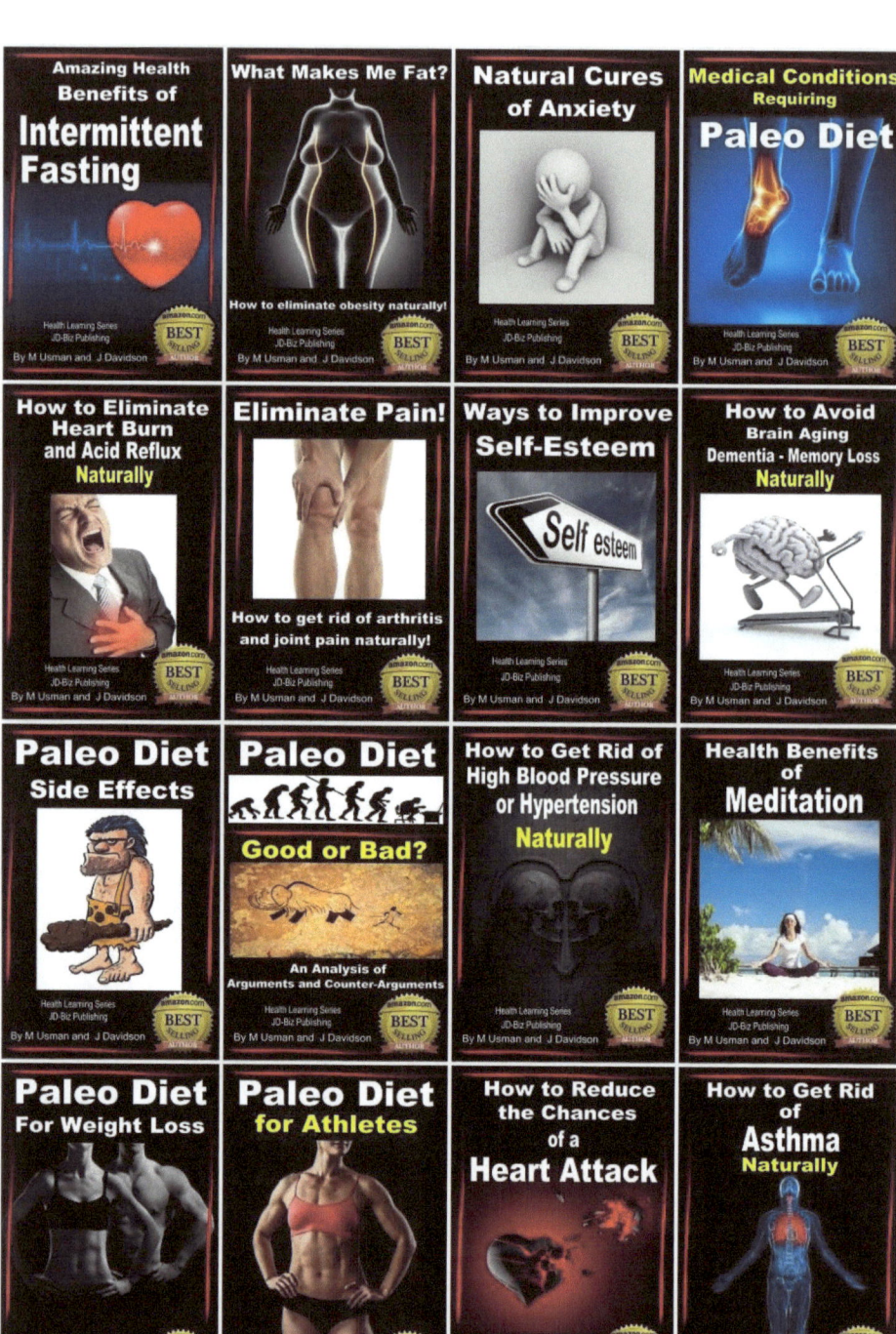

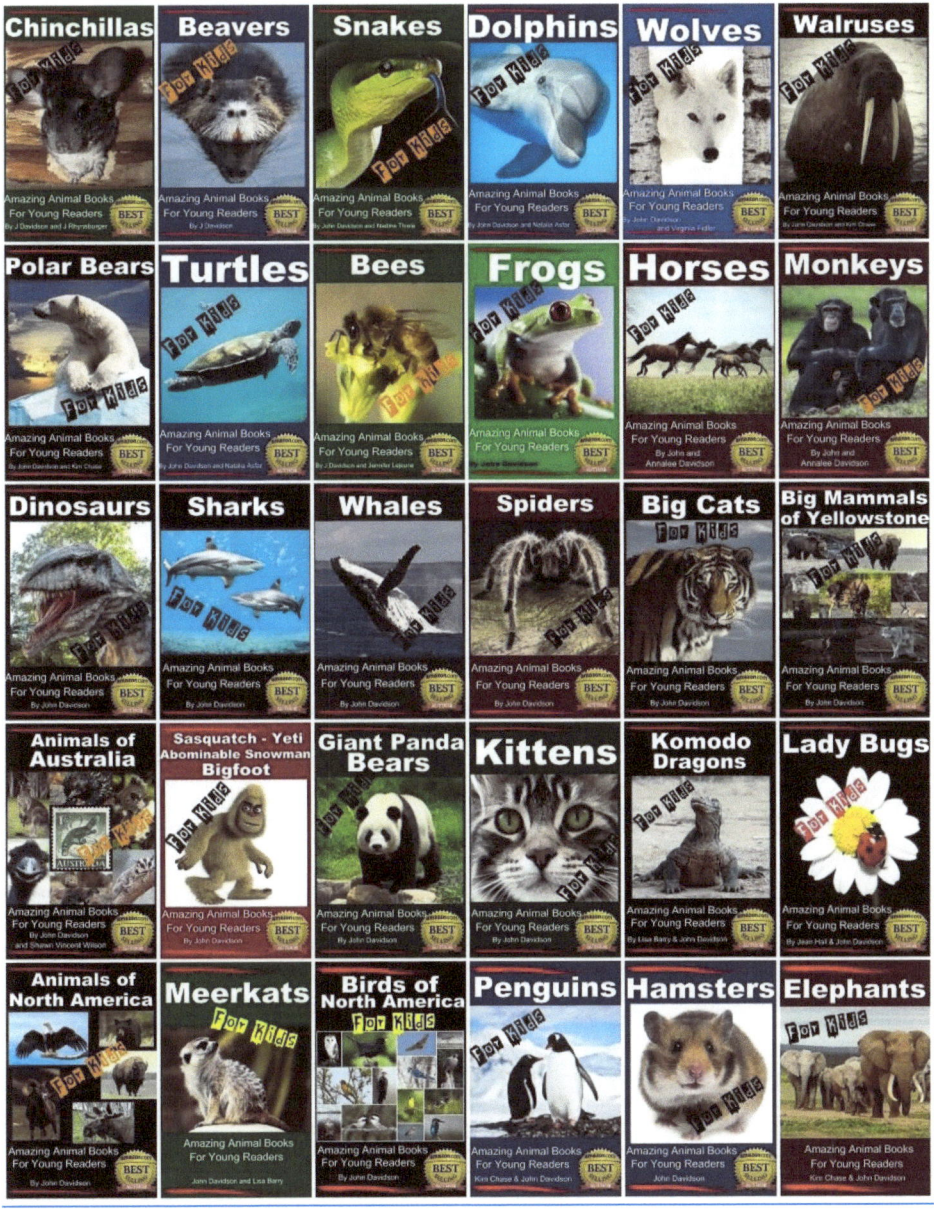

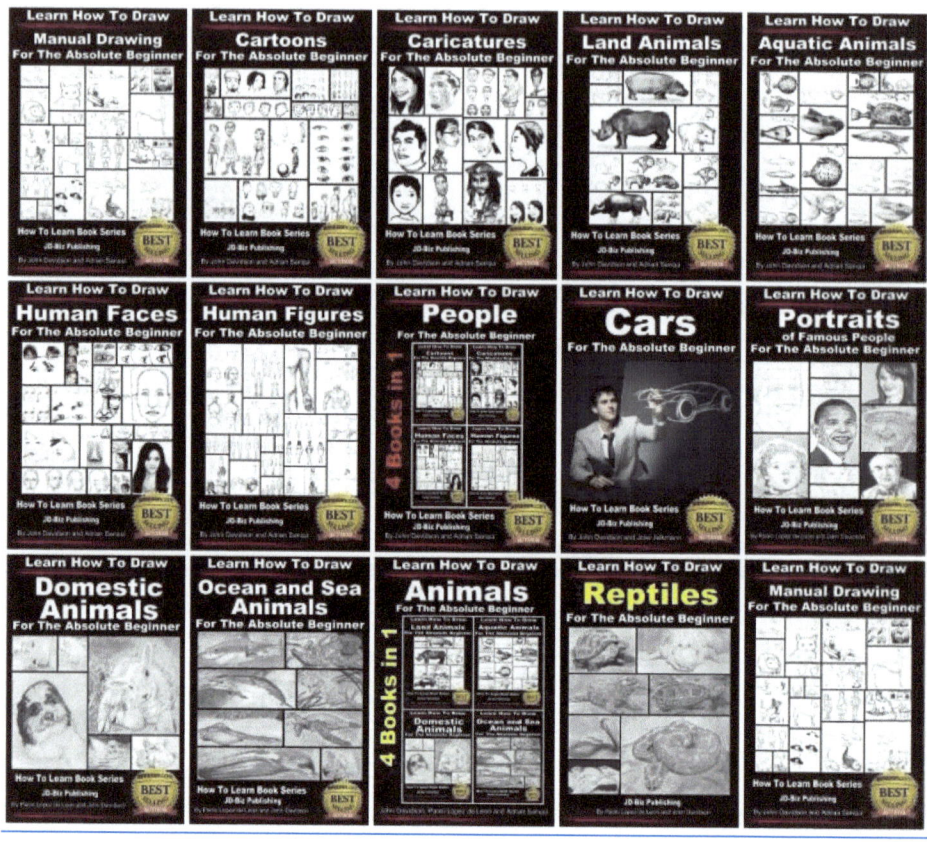

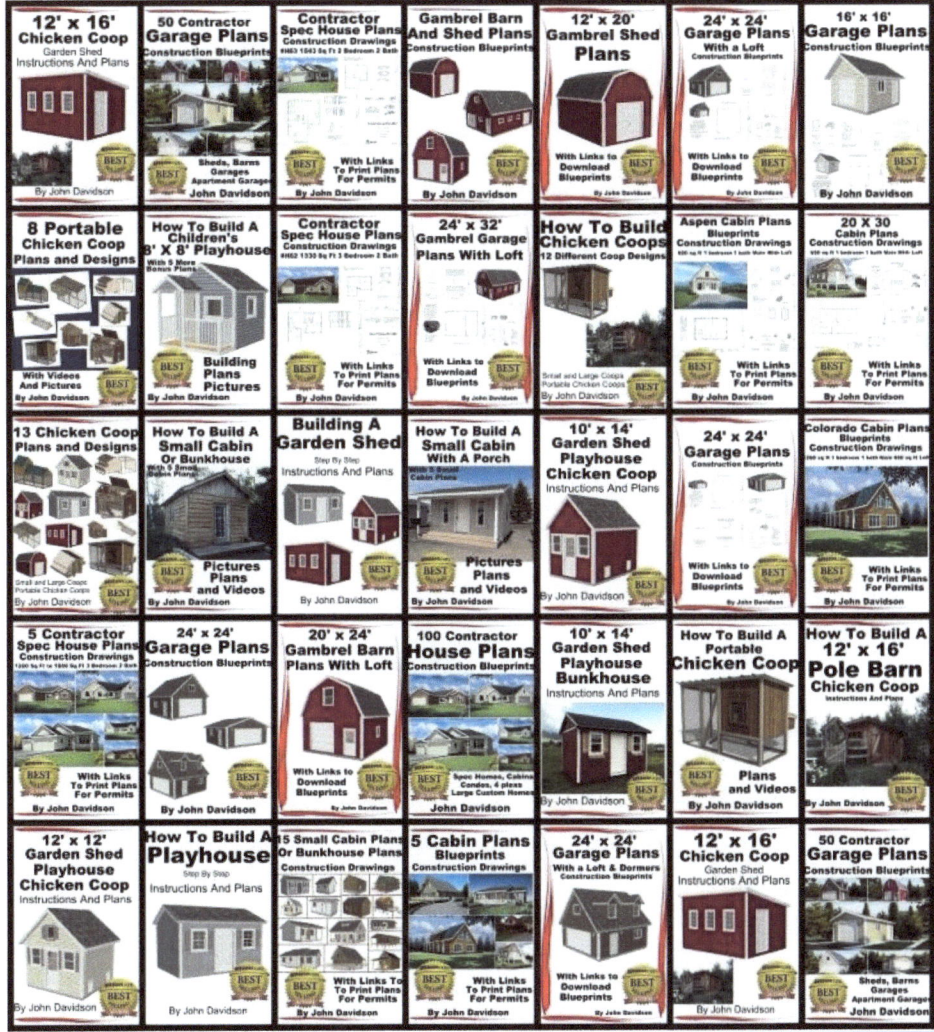

Check out some of the Entrepreneur Series books

Entrepreneur Series books on Amazon

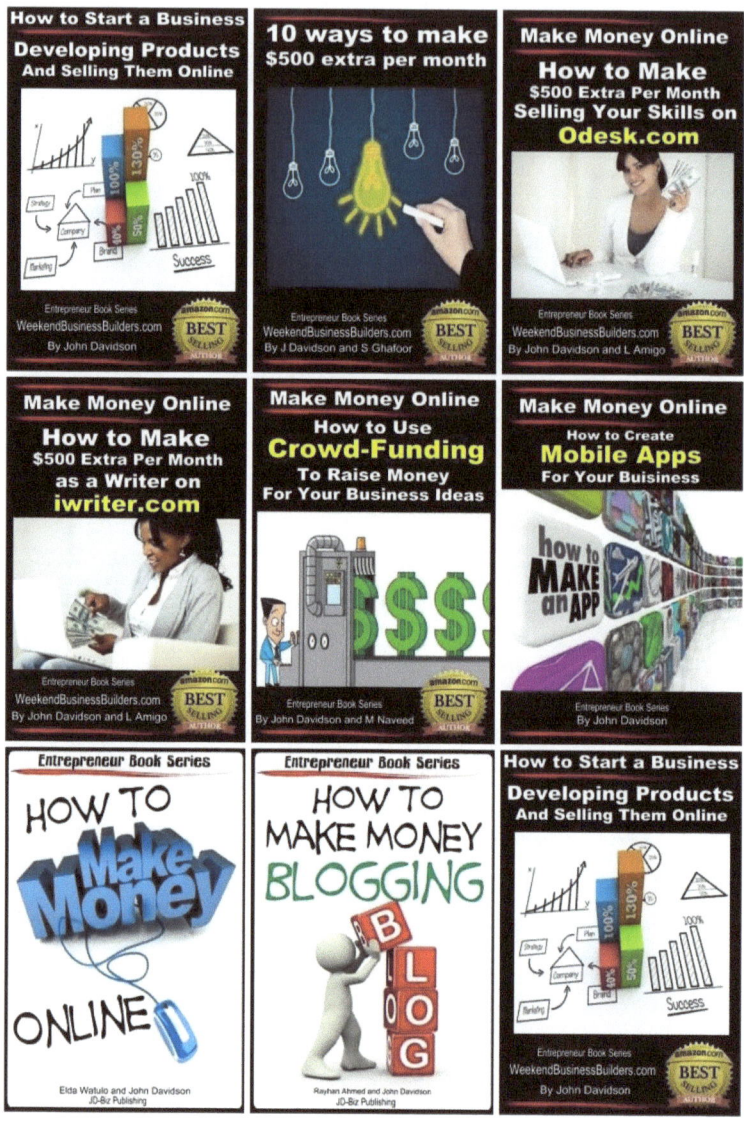

Our books are available at

1. Amazon.com

2. Barnes and Noble

3. Itunes

4. Kobo

5. Smashwords

6. Google Play Books

Download Free Books!

http://MendonCottageBooks.com

Publisher

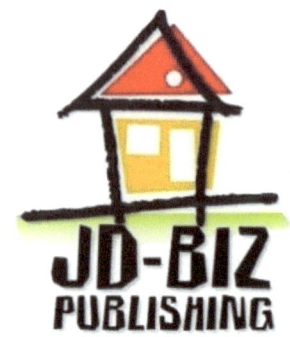

JD-Biz Corp

P O Box 374

Mendon, Utah 84325

http://www.jd-biz.com/

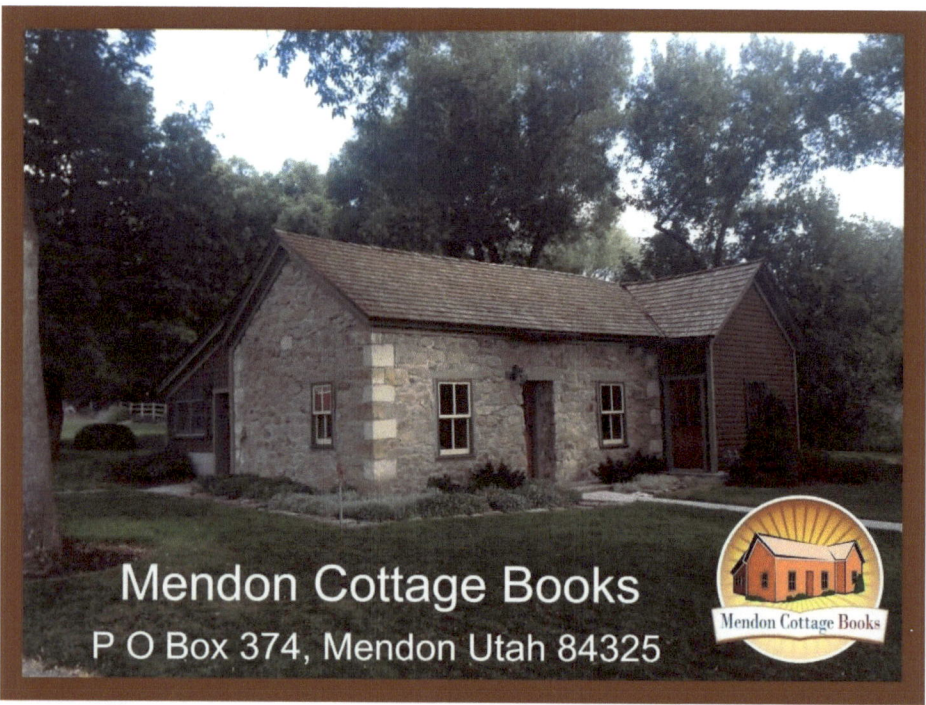

www.ingramcontent.com/pod-product-compliance
Lightning Source LLC
Chambersburg PA
CBHW050820290526
45792CB00001B/202